Distribution, publication, and copying in any form are prohibited and subject to damages.

TEN HYPNOSES

Copying, publishing, and sharing with third parties are only permitted with the written consent of the author. Please observe the notes on copyright and usage.

Distribution, publication, and copying in any form are prohibited and subject to damages.

Copying, publishing, and sharing with third parties are only permitted with the written consent of the author. Please observe the notes on copyright and usage.

Distribution, publication, and copying in any form are prohibited and subject to damages.

Ingo Michael Simon

TEN HYPNOSES

19

ADDICTION TENDENCIES

Copying, publishing, and sharing with third parties are only permitted with the written consent of the author. Please observe the notes on copyright and usage.

Distribution, publication, and copying in any form are prohibited and subject to damages.

© 2024 Ingo Michael Simon
All rights reserved.
Independently published
www.ingosimon.com

Important Notes for Urgent Attention:
The contents of this book are based on the practical experiences of the author with hypnosis applications and psychotherapy in a trance state. Although the author has strived for the utmost care, errors or misunderstandings in the presentation cannot be completely excluded. Therapeutic work with people and the application of hypnosis are solely the responsibility of the hypnotist. It cannot be ruled out that parts of this book may be misunderstood or that the application of a presented procedure may cause an undesirable reaction in the client. The author also assumes no co-responsibility if work with a client is carried out with reference to the statements in this book.

The Author:
Ingo Michael Simon studied psychology and education and is a hypnotherapist with practices in southwestern Germany and Switzerland. With the help of hypnosis-supported psychotherapy, he primarily treats people with persistent psychological conditions. His practice focuses on anxiety disorders, pathological compulsions, and psychosomatic illnesses. His therapeutic offerings mainly include classical and modern hypnosis applications and the dreamland therapy he developed himself.

Copying, publishing, and sharing with third parties are only permitted with the written consent of the author. Please observe the notes on copyright and usage.

Distribution, publication, and copying in any form are prohibited and subject to damages.

Notes on Copyright and Usage

Copying, publishing, and sharing with third parties is prohibited and only permitted with the written consent of the author. Please observe the following copyright and usage guidelines.

This work has been carefully crafted and created to the best of the author's knowledge and personal experience. It comprises text templates and application guidelines for professional hypnosis sessions. The author is a licensed psychotherapist with extensive experience in psychotherapy, coaching, and personal training using hypnotic techniques and methods. Nevertheless, the author and the publisher assume no liability for the accuracy of information, instructions, and advice, nor for any typographical errors. The author and publisher accept no responsibility or liability for the application of these texts and recommendations with clients or patients, nor for any potential consequences or unexpected reactions. It is expressly noted that the application of therapeutic and advisory techniques and formulations lies solely and entirely within the responsibility of the practitioner. This also applies to adherence to the boundaries of legally regulated medical and therapeutic practices. The fact that a book containing action proposals is freely available for sale does not imply that its application with clients or patients is permitted for everyone.

Distribution, publication, and copying in any form are prohibited and subject to damages.

Copying, publishing, and sharing with third parties are only permitted with the written consent of the author. Please observe the notes on copyright and usage.

Distribution, publication, and copying in any form are prohibited and subject to damages.

Table of Contents

Introduction 9

#1 11

#2 16

#3 22

#4 28

#5 34

#6 39

#7 44

#8 49

#9 55

#10 60

Overview of All Titles in the Series "Ten Hypnoses" 65

Copying, publishing, and sharing with third parties are only permitted with the written consent of the author. Please observe the notes on copyright and usage.

Distribution, publication, and copying in any form are prohibited and subject to damages.

Copying, publishing, and sharing with third parties are only permitted with the written consent of the author. Please observe the notes on copyright and usage.

Introduction

The series "Ten Hypnoses" is very well known in Germany, Austria, and Switzerland as a collection of texts for therapeutic work and is used by numerous psychotherapeutic practices, doctors, therapists, coaches, and other helping professionals. I am pleased to now be able to offer these texts in other countries as well.

Most therapists have their own methods for inducing and deepening trance as well as for exiting trance. Therefore, I have focused on the main part of the hypnosis. The texts in this book can be integrated as the main part into any hypnosis process.

The texts in this collection use various hypnosis techniques. I will not explain these in detail, as I assume that users have the appropriate training. It is also not necessary to understand the exact structure or functioning of the different parts. The texts can simply be read aloud, and they will have their effect.

Decide for yourself which text best suits your client or patient at any given time. You can also combine passages from different texts. It is not about using all ten hypnoses in sequence. It is a selection of possibilities.

I want to emphasize that books cannot replace therapy. Psychotherapy or other therapeutic treatments involve much more. A careful diagnosis is the necessary basis for deciding on the use of methods, including whether hypnosis or one of my texts should be used. Even in this case, preparatory discussions, follow-up discussions during the session, and of course, a therapeutic concept for the sequence of sessions and the content approaches are essential parts of therapy. This cannot and should not be achieved with a collection of texts.

In any case, I wish you much success in your work and I am pleased if my text templates can contribute in a small way.

Ingo Michael Simon

#1

You've realized that alcohol served a certain function for you that you don't actually need ... ... Drinking sometimes brought you short-term relief and a bit of calm ... ... but you know that alcohol creates more problems than it can truly solve ... ... You have decided to tackle all your problems without alcohol because that's something you can really do ... ... Problems can be solved entirely without alcohol ... ... You are so strong that you can resolve your issues from within yourself and by your own strength ... ... It's truly remarkable how much you succeed in abstaining from alcohol in this moment ... ... and equally remarkable and strong that you anchor this attitude deep within yourself ... ... By your own decision to simply leave alcohol behind ... ... you realize that your inner power and strength are entirely sufficient to manage your problems ... ... and also to be in a good mood and relax ... ... For that, you have much better options than drinking alcohol ... ... You succeed in finding calm ... ... When you pay attention to your body now ... ... you feel deep and pleasant relaxation at this moment ... ...

You are relaxing right now, completely without alcohol ... ... and it was very easy for you to reach this wonderful state of rest and stay calm ... ... You can do even more, completely free from alcohol ... ... At this moment, you can relax even deeper, just because you want to ... ... So, relax now even more and convince yourself that you can come to rest entirely without alcohol, just like now ... ... exactly like now ... ... By convincing yourself now that you can relax completely without alcohol, you recognize that you never needed alcohol ... ... You never needed alcohol ... ... and you will never need alcohol ... ... You will never need alcohol ... ... Alcohol becomes almost meaningless ... ... completely indifferent ...

... ... Even in the company of others, alcohol remains completely meaningless to you ... ... You don't even consider drinking in social settings because you prefer to be cheerful and clear-headed ... ... just like now ... ... If you now examine or follow your own thoughts, you can quickly realize that your thoughts are completely clear and pure ... ... Every thought you observe is precise and clear ... ... and you prefer this clarity of thought above all else ... ... It's truly remarkable how quickly you can internalize this and how quickly you can now switch to clarity of thought by abstaining from alcohol ... ... You completely abstain from alcohol ... ... You completely abstain from alcohol from now on ... ... But what exactly are you abstaining from? ... ... You are abstaining from drunkenness that threw you off balance ... ... You are abstaining from foggy and slow thoughts ... ... You are abstaining from all the harmful effects of alcohol ... ... You are only giving up the damaging influences of alcohol ... ... By doing so, you gain so much good in return ... ... You regain the unrestricted clarity of your thoughts ... ... You regain health and strength ... ... You gain a healthier and freer life ... ... You gain a truly healthier and much freer life ... ... and this gain strengthens your resolve to leave alcohol behind and be and remain completely free from alcohol ... ... You want to be free from alcohol and stay free from it ... ... Your decision is firm ... ... Your decision for a healthier and freer life ... ... without alcohol ... ... completely without alcohol ... ... Your decision is unshakeable and stable ... ... Nothing and no one can shake your resolve ... ... nothing and no one, because you made this decision with the clarity of your thoughts ... ... You decided with the clarity of your thoughts ... ... never again alcohol ... ... never again alcohol ...

... ... In fact, you don't have to break the habit of drinking, because that has already happened ... ... You are a non-drinker ... ... You are anti-alcohol ... ... You have already stopped drinking ... ... So you don't have to stop drinking ... ... Any reach for alcohol would be starting again, which is out of the question for you ... ... You will never start drinking alcohol again ... ... You are already free from alcohol and will remain permanently free from it ... ... You are already dry and will remain permanently dry ... ... You are already anti-alcohol and will remain anti-alcohol ... ... You have stopped drinking ... ... Isn't it remarkable that you now realize that you have actually already stopped? ... ... Make it clear to yourself ... ... You have already stopped drinking ... ... and you will not start again ... ... You don't need to take the step of stopping, because you have already done it ... ... You have already quit ... ... stopped drinking ... ... Your decision to never drink alcohol again was made a long time ago ... ... Your decision to never drink alcohol again is firm now ... ... unshakably firm ... ... Your decision to never drink alcohol again will remain firm ... ... You are almost stubborn and relentless when it comes to alcohol ... ... a stubborn anti-alcohol person ... ... In your decision to never drink alcohol again, you are more stubborn than ever before ... ... because your decision was and is firm ... ... Your decision is truly rock-solid ... ... never again alcohol ... ... You align your entire organism to this ... ... Your whole body follows this will and this decision ... ... Very soon, you won't even be able to imagine that you ever drank alcohol ... ... because alcohol will become meaningless to you ... ... completely meaningless ...

Your organism is now adjusting to living without alcohol forever ... ... In your waking everyday life, it's like this: just the sight of alcoholic beverages makes you feel aversion ... ... Just the sight of a glass of beer or wine or any other alcoholic drink makes you recoil and not want anything to do with alcohol ... ... The smell of alcoholic beverages immediately reminds you that your decision is firm ... ... Leave alcohol behind ... ... Leave alcohol behind ... ... If you detect an alcoholic taste, for example in food, you immediately feel the impulse to leave that food ... ... Anything that smells or tastes like alcohol, looks like it, or feels like it, is your signal to leave it ... ... You leave alcohol behind ... ... forever ... ... because you are free from alcohol and will stay free from alcohol ... ... You are and remain free ...

#2

You have made an important decision ... ... You have decided never to drink alcohol again ... ... That is a good and right decision because it means you have chosen health and freedom ... ... Earlier, you thought alcohol could open up new possibilities for you, but it only narrowed your options ... ... today you know that ... ... Today, you understand that you can only truly be free without alcohol ... ... and that is your goal ... ... to be free and to remain free ... ... free from alcohol ... ... and to stay free from alcohol ... ... Earlier, you also thought that alcohol could be enjoyable, but now you know that this was also an illusion ... ... Alcohol was no enjoyment for you ... ... You associate alcohol with drunkenness and a hangover the next day ... ... You have also experienced how it feels when you get sick from drinking alcohol ... ... or suddenly felt the urge to drink more or to drink in the morning ... ... That was pure nausea ... ... You know what it's like to feel sick from alcohol ... ... You remember this feeling ... ... more than that ... ... Your body remembers it and wants to avoid any nausea caused by alcohol from now on ... ... If you now imagine exactly how it felt when you got sick ... ... you can develop an even stronger will never to drink alcohol again ... ... Alcohol repulses you ... ... You completely reject these drinks that only bring nausea and illness ... ... At the thought of alcohol, you immediately think of nausea ... ... Both are now inseparable and forever connected ... ... Alcohol and nausea ... ... Alcohol and nausea ... ... This connection is ingrained in your memory ... ... Alcohol and nausea ... ... This connection is ingrained in your feelings ... ... Alcohol and nausea ... ... and more than that ... ... The connection of alcohol with the feeling of nausea becomes a sentence ... ... a new belief for you ... ... Alcohol only brings nausea ... ... This sentence is deeply ingrained in your belief ... ... Alcohol only brings nausea ... ... It is deeply ingrained in your body feeling ... ... Alcohol only brings nausea ...

... ... Your new attitude towards alcohol creates a resistance within you ... ... a resistance that immediately arises when you might come into contact with alcohol ... ... You feel this resistance because you reject alcohol ... ... You reject alcohol ... ... You rigorously reject alcohol ... ... The mere idea of drinking alcohol repulses you ... ... Everything in you rebels at the thought of drinking alcohol ... ... Every fiber of your body rebels at the idea of drinking alcohol ... ... At the thought of alcohol, you can only feel disgust and revulsion ... ... The thought of drinking is downright unpleasant to you ... ... Right now, you can deeply embed this thought within yourself ... ... because your entire body is aligning with you to associate alcohol with revulsion and disgust ... ... So, your body will also resist any association with alcohol ... ... Your body completely rejects alcohol because alcohol is disgusting ... ... Alcohol is disgusting ... ... Alcohol is truly disgusting ... ... Your body helps you to recognize this again and again ... ... your body shows you repeatedly that it does not want any alcohol ... ... Your body shows you again and again that it completely rejects alcohol ... ... But your thoughts also reject alcohol ... ... Your mind knows that alcohol is unpleasant ... ... downright disgusting because alcohol makes you sick ... ... Alcohol only brings nausea ... ... Alcohol truly only brings nausea ... ... Your thoughts follow the wisdom of your mind, which knows for sure that alcohol only has harmful effects ... ... Your thoughts follow the wisdom of your mind, which is certain that alcohol only brings nausea ...

... ... Today marks the beginning of a new and healthier chapter in your life because you have stopped drinking ... ... You have already stopped, and today you make clear to yourself what benefits this has for you ... ... because you never have to endure nausea from alcohol again ... ... Your thoughts will never be clouded by alcohol again ... ... From now on, you can always think and feel clearly at all times ... ... without alcohol ... ... think clearly without alcohol ... ... as clear as now because now you are free from alcohol ... ... and this state is the most valuable you can experience ... ... You now focus on the clarity of your thoughts, and in doing so, your revulsion to alcohol grows stronger ... ... Your revulsion to alcohol grows stronger ... ... so strong that you can hardly imagine that you ever enjoyed drinking ... ... Enjoying drinking is unimaginable ... ... drinking is absolutely unimaginable ... ... At the thought of drinking alcohol, you already feel the strong revulsion ... ... the rejection ... ... because you reject alcohol ... ... You strictly reject alcohol ... ... You feel revulsion at the thought of alcohol ... ... a very strong revulsion that grows and becomes more stable with every thought and consideration ... ... Every time you think of alcohol or consider drinking, your rejection grows ... ... because you strictly reject alcohol ...

... ... Even in social settings, it is very easy for you to leave alcohol behind ... ... because just the sight of alcoholic beverages awakens your revulsion and rejection ... ... Every glass that could be filled with alcoholic beverages makes you feel your deep rejection ... ... You will never drink alcohol again ... ... never drink alcohol again ... ... and if alcohol is offered to you, your revulsion is even stronger ... ... so strong that you immediately reject it ... ... so strong that you immediately reject it ...

Your entire inner being is now adjusting to rejecting alcohol forever and feeling a strong aversion to alcohol ... ... In your waking everyday life, it's like this: just the sight of alcoholic beverages makes you feel this disgust ... ... Just the sight of a glass of beer or wine or any other alcoholic drink makes you feel only revulsion and disgust and not want anything to do with alcohol ... ... The smell of alcoholic beverages evokes disgust and rejection in you ... ... If you detect an alcoholic taste, for example in food, you immediately feel sick and leave the food ... ... Anything that smells or tastes like alcohol, looks like it, or feels like it, evokes your revulsion and disgust for alcohol ... ... You leave alcohol behind ... ... forever ... ... because you are free from alcohol and will stay free from alcohol ... ... You are and remain free ...

#3

The following version of a hypnosis main part works with an anchor in the form of a handy note with the printed words "Never Again Alcohol." An anchor is a trigger that creates a certain feeling or thought. We want to help the client adjust to letting go faster with the help of a "reminder card" when they notice in everyday life that the past is influencing their actions. We discuss this with the client before the session and prepare the reminder card. It can be a labeled business card or something similar. The card is prepared and given to the client to hold loosely in their hand during the hypnosis or place on their body, for example, on the solar plexus. The card should be carried by the client after the hypnosis, in their pants pocket or jacket pocket.

You have made a clear decision to never drink alcohol again ... ... To send alcohol to the place of the past and leave it there forever ... ... because that's where alcohol belongs, in the past ... ... You will always remember the time of drinking, the harmful and destructive effect of alcohol, but now it's over ... ... because the present belongs to you alone ... ... there is no more room for alcohol in your life ... ... It was your own holding on that allowed alcohol to control your life so much, but that had to be ... ... back then it couldn't be any different, but today it can be different ... ... today it really can be different ... ... You have reached a very special point ... ... You have processed and understood ... ... Therefore, now is the right time to let go of alcohol once and for all ... ... Never again alcohol ... ... that is your motto ... ... Never again alcohol ... ... Your creed ... ... Never again alcohol ...

... ... You have decided that you want to let go of alcohol ... ... You have understood that it is you who must make absolute truth out of your intentions ... ... You know that it is you who creates your success ... ... and you are ready to do so ... ... You are ready to give everything necessary to free yourself from alcohol once and for all ... ... You have the potential ... ... you have the strength you need ... ... But you want more ... ... You want to be able to fully utilize your traits and abilities at all times ... ... You want to be able to let go of any thought of alcohol anytime and immediately ... ... especially if you ever think about drinking again ... ... and you can do that ... ... let go immediately ... ... You know the right attitude ... ... Never again alcohol ... ... It is like a message to yourself ... ... Never again alcohol ... ... It is like a reminder ... ... Never again alcohol ... ... like a command that only you can give yourself ... ... Never again alcohol ...

You have a card with exactly this inscription, the card bears your task ... ... Never again alcohol ... ... You now feel this inner strength growing within you ... ... You know that you can achieve anything ... ... your will and readiness grow with every breath and with every breath it becomes clearer ... ... Never again alcohol ... ... The card shows it to you every day ... ... It shows you your attitude that you can carry with you always ... ... Never again alcohol ... ... It helps you become stronger every day and finally to be and stay free ... ... Whenever the slightest doubt arises within you, you immediately take the card in your hand and read the inscription clearly, you look at it ... ... Never again alcohol ... ... Then you immediately feel the effect, you feel that this is your truth ... ... You do this every day ... ... You simply let go of the alcohol ... ... You simply let go of the alcohol ...

The card shows it to you every day ... ... It shows you your own attitude that you can carry with you always ... ... It helps you through difficult moments ... ... Whenever the slightest doubt arises within you, you immediately take the card in your hand and look at it ... ... Never again alcohol ... ... Then you immediately feel the effect, you feel that this is your truth ...

... ... Now consciously take your reminder card in your hand ... ... Hold it tightly ... ... Have you noticed that you are holding onto something again? ... ... This time you are holding onto freedom ... ... and as incredible and paradoxical as it may sound ... ... This is a good kind of holding on ... ... holding on to your goal of being and staying free from alcohol ... ... holding on to the fact that you are important to yourself ... ... holding on to your goal of freeing yourself from alcohol forever ... ... holding on to the fact that there is nothing more important to you than finally letting go of alcohol ... ... that there is nothing more important than living without alcohol ... ... completely without alcohol ... ... what is over, you let go of, and the time of alcohol is now over ... ... The time of alcohol is now really and finally over ... ... The card you feel between your fingers reminds you of this

... ... it helps you let go of alcohol ... ... it helps you be free and stay free ... ... it helps you with your new and healthy life completely without alcohol ...

... ... [Now instruct the client to open their eyes and read the inscription on the card in trance. This enhances the effect. Opening the eyes is a fractionation, but can be done without a specific announcement or counting. Anyone can open their eyes in trance. In a stable and deep trance, it is somewhat difficult because the client is tired and sluggish. Simply stay with the suggestive request until the eyes open and the card is read. If you prefer to initiate fractionation by counting steps, you can do that of course. It is not necessary.] ... ...

... ... Consciously feel the reminder card between your fingers and, if you want, briefly open your eyes and look at the card ... ... open your eyes and read what is written there ... ... Never again alcohol ... ... You can recognize these words ... ... Never again alcohol ... ... This card only says what you yourself have decided, what corresponds to your own decision and your will ... ... Never again alcohol ... ... Now close your eyes again and let the words you have read sink deeply within you ... ... very deeply ...

You still feel the card between your fingers ... ... You know that it will remind you every day that you are and remain free from alcohol ... ... Whenever you take the card in your hand and read it, you immediately feel more free and calm inside ... ... you immediately feel that your life without alcohol is much freer and more beautiful ... ... Whenever you carry the card with you, you feel calmer and freer inside ... ... calmer and freer ... ... It happens naturally because your inner self knows that this card reminds you of what you have done today ... ... your liberation from alcohol ...

#4

The following version of a hypnosis main part works with an anchor in the form of a handy note with an affirmation: "I now take back control of my needs and take responsibility for my health. I can and will turn away from alcohol forever." An anchor is a trigger that creates a certain feeling or thought. We want to help the client adjust to letting go faster with the help of a "reminder card" when they notice in everyday life that the past is influencing their actions. We discuss this with the client before the session and prepare the reminder card. It can be a labeled business card or something similar. The card is prepared and given to the client to hold loosely in their hand during the hypnosis or place on their body, for example, on the solar plexus. The card should be carried by the client after the hypnosis, in their pants pocket or jacket pocket.

You have stopped drinking alcohol ... ... That was a wise and prudent decision because you have chosen a healthier and freer life ... ... Alcohol now belongs to the past ... ... and you will never want to start drinking again ... ... never let alcohol control your life again, because now and in the future only you decide ... ... Only you alone decide what can be in your life ... ... and alcohol can never be part of it again ... ... Your decision is firm and unchangeable ... ... You avoid alcohol like poison ... ... because alcohol is poison for your body and poison for your mind ... ... You will never again allow alcohol to cloud your mind and poison your body because you avoid alcohol for all time ... ... You know it is right to avoid alcohol because you know the harmful effects alcohol has ... ... You know the effects of alcohol that have only brought you harm ... ... You also know that you can satisfy your needs completely without alcohol ... ... because by drinking alcohol you neglected your true needs ... ... you just numbed yourself and couldn't pay attention to what you really needed ... ... Alcohol was taking control ... ... But you will not allow that ... ... You now take control of your life yourself ... ... You now take control of your needs yourself ... ... You take responsibility for your life ... ... Alcohol only brings you harm ... ... But you want to be healthy ... ... You have a right to health, and that is best achieved without alcohol ... ... You turn away from alcohol ... ... It's like a creed that you fully adopt ... ... You have found your creed, and it is written on your card ... ... So you can carry it with you like a prayer and always strengthen yourself with your own belief ... ... Deep within you, these words work that you speak with me in your thoughts ... ... and if you want, speak them aloud or whisper them so you can hear and feel them ... ... You say ...

I now take back control of my needs and take responsibility for my health. I can and will turn away from alcohol forever.

That is what counts because that is your decision ... ... Your creed, which you deeply internalize ... ... Your commitment to yourself ... ... to your own belief ... ... to your decision ... ... to your firm will ... ... to your path ... ... Once again you say ...

I now take back control of my needs and take responsibility for my health. I can and will turn away from alcohol forever.

... ... good ... ... very good ... ... You know what matters, and you know that this attitude can and will accompany you forever because you have decided to let go of alcohol forever ... ... and whether you are alone or in company, you stick to it ... ... You avoid alcohol for a self-determined life ... ... You avoid alcohol for a healthy life ... ... You avoid alcohol for a responsible life ... ... You avoid alcohol for yourself ... ... You do this for yourself because you are worth avoiding alcohol ... ... avoiding it forever ... ... and you have help ... ... great help in your everyday life ... ... You have the card that is a reminder card for you ... ... a card that reminds you of your own decision ... ... helps you to always reassure yourself that you can manage to avoid alcohol forever ... ... to stay strong and steadfast and never succumb to temptation ... ... because alcohol is no longer a temptation for you ... ... Alcohol is over ... ... Your card reminds you of this ... ... You can read it whenever you want and thereby strengthen your resolve ... ... Your attitude becomes a firm belief ... ... a prayer and a truth ... ... because you establish it today ... ... You carry your belief card in your hand, can feel it, and you know what is written on it ...

... ... [Now instruct the client to open their eyes and read the inscription on the card in trance. This enhances the effect. Opening the eyes is a fractionation, but can be done without a specific announcement or counting. Anyone can open their eyes in trance. In a stable and deep trance, it is somewhat difficult because the client is tired and sluggish. Simply stay with the suggestive request until the eyes open and the card is read. If you prefer to initiate fractionation by counting steps, you can do that of course. It is not necessary.] ... ...

... ... Consciously feel the card between your fingers and open your eyes briefly and look at the card ... ... open your eyes and read what is written there ... ... I now take back control of my needs and take responsibility for my health. I can and will turn away from alcohol forever ... ... You can clearly recognize these words ... ... This card only says what you yourself have decided, what corresponds to your own decision and your will ... ... Let's read together once more what is written there ... ... I now take back control of my needs and take responsibility for my health. I can and will turn away from alcohol forever ... ... Now close your eyes again and let the words you have read sink deeply within you ... ... very deeply ...

Carry this card with you always ... ... put it in your pocket so it can work its effect throughout the day ... ... because whenever you carry this card with you, it is a confirmation that you continue your path without alcohol ... ... just by putting the card in your pocket, you actively and consciously decide to avoid alcohol forever ... ... and whenever you take the card in your hand and read what is written on it, your resolve becomes firmer and more stable ... ... You avoid alcohol ...

#5

You are fed up with drinking ... ... in fact, you don't want to drink anything anymore and you don't need to drink alcohol ... ... You are truly fed up ... ... satisfied and you don't need alcohol anymore ... ... your mind knows this and keeps repeating it ... ... I don't need alcohol and I don't want alcohol ... ... I don't need alcohol and I don't want alcohol ... ... I don't need alcohol and I don't want alcohol ... ... and what your mind knows and understands can become your truth as soon as your entire organism has also understood it ... ... Today is that day ... ... this special day when your organism has fully understood that it's time to stop drinking alcohol ... ... And now it's about making sure that your deep inner self, the world of your moods and feelings, can take the same step ... ... and it's easier than you thought ... ... Perhaps you're wondering how exactly it can happen that your subconscious takes the same step as your mind ... ... Maybe you're wondering how quickly it can happen that your subconscious fully adjusts to being an anti-alcohol person from now on ... ... and when you think about it carefully, you surely ask yourself what your subconscious can do for you once it has decided that you will leave alcohol behind once and for all and never drink alcohol again ... ... There is a clear and definite answer for you ... ... Your subconscious can and will protect you by strictly rejecting alcohol ... ... Even if your mind would think about how it would be to drink alcohol again, your subconscious will take complete control and not allow the drinking of alcohol anymore ... ... That's what your subconscious can do and that's what it will do ... ... You just have to do one thing ... ... just one thing, which I will help you with now ... ... You have to replace the image of alcohol with a new one ... ... The truly amazing thing is that replacing alcohol is incredibly easy ... ... So let's start by opening the door to your subconscious to make you an anti-alcohol person ... ... now ... ... right now ...

... ... Imagine a large bottle of alcohol in front of your inner eye ... ... maybe with the alcoholic drink you drank the most ... ... a huge bottle that can hold ten liters ... ... Imagine it ... ... filled to the top ... ... good ... ... That's how the image should look ... ... and now we start changing the image ... ... Imagine the bottle is slowly being emptied ... ...

but keep it upright ... ... Just look at the image and imagine that the level in the bottle is slowly going down ... ... as if someone had opened a valve or pulled the plug of a bathtub ... ... Connect this with your breathing ... ... Imagine that the level in the bottle goes down a bit with each exhale ... ... Every time you exhale, the level in the bottle drops because it's draining ... ... and with each inhale, you gain strength for the next step ...

... ... [Speak the following suggestions always during the client's exhale and exhale clearly while speaking. This extends the process of exhaling and suggests the draining of alcohol from the bottle!] ... ...

... ... Exhale and let the level drop ... ... good ... ...

... ... The level drops deeper and deeper ... ... excellent ...

... ... The level in the bottle drops ... ... very good ... ...

... ... Alcohol sinks slowly ... ... You see it clearly ... ...

... ... The alcohol sinks ... ... You can feel it ... ...

... ... The alcohol disappears from the bottle ... ... and you become free ... ...

...... The alcohol disappears from your body ...... and you become free ......

...... The bottle eventually empties ...... Now ......

...... The bottle is completely empty ...... Now ......

...... You are free from alcohol ...... Now ......

...... free ...... completely free ......

...... [Now continue "normally"] ......

Breathe calmly and relaxed and look at the image of the empty bottle ...... Your subconscious imprints this deeply ...... You no longer have the need to drink alcohol because the need has disappeared ...... You have erased it, changed the inner image ...... The thought of alcohol is now equivalent to the image of a large empty bottle ...... Each breath empties this bottle ...... Any thought of filling it again is immediately interrupted by your subconscious, as it empties this notion with just one breath ...... Whenever you think about how drinking alcohol could be, your subconscious empties this thought ...... because there is no more alcohol in your inner self ...... The image of the draining bottle makes drinking alcohol impossible ...... absolutely impossible because you can no longer feel the need for alcohol ...

This change happens deep within you ... ... in the world of your emotions, because that's where your subconscious resides, which makes any thought of alcohol disappear just like the alcohol from your bottle ... ... Whenever you think of alcohol, your subconscious empties the desire for alcohol immediately

... ... Whenever you see alcoholic beverages, your subconscious empties the desire for alcohol immediately ... ... Whenever you smell or taste alcohol, your subconscious empties the desire for alcohol immediately ... ... Whenever you think of alcohol, your subconscious empties this thought immediately ... ... You are free from alcohol ... ... free ... ... completely free ... ...

You have stopped drinking alcohol ... ... in fact, you don't want to drink anything anymore and you don't need to drink alcohol ... ... You have stopped ... ... You don't need alcohol anymore ... ... your mind knows this and keeps repeating it ... ... I don't need alcohol and I don't want alcohol ... ... I don't need alcohol and I don't want alcohol ... ... I don't need alcohol and I don't want alcohol ... ... and what your mind knows and understands can become your truth as soon as your entire organism has also understood it ... ... Today is that day ... ... this special day when your organism has fully understood that you don't need alcohol and can replace it with something new ... ... something healthy and creative ... ... And now it's about creating new images within you ... ... and that is much easier than you could have imagined ... ... Perhaps you're wondering how exactly it can happen that your subconscious takes the same step as your mind ... ... Maybe you're wondering how quickly it can happen that your subconscious fully adjusts to leaving the drinking behind and engaging in more interesting activities ... ... and when you think about it carefully, you surely ask yourself what your subconscious can do for you once it has decided to let new creative images arise and never drink alcohol again ... ... There is a clear and definite answer for you ... ... Your subconscious can and will help you by always replacing alcohol with a new image ... ... always replacing it with another need ... ... Even if your mind would think about how it would be to drink alcohol again, your subconscious will take complete control and not allow the drinking of alcohol anymore ... ... That's what your subconscious can do and that's what it will do ... ... You just have to do one thing ... ... just one thing, which I will help you with now ... ... You have to replace the image of alcohol with a new one ... ... The truly amazing thing is that replacing alcohol is incredibly easy ... ... So let's start by opening the door to your subconscious to make you an anti-alcohol person ... ... now ... ... right now ...

... ... Imagine a large empty bottle in front of your inner eye ... ... Since you no longer need alcohol and completely reject alcohol, this bottle is completely empty today ... ... You have already emptied it by deciding to stop drinking alcohol ... ... In front of you stands a huge empty bottle that can hold ten liters ... ... Imagine it ... ... completely empty ... ... good ... ... That's how the image should look ... ... and now we start changing the image ... ... Imagine the bottle is slowly being filled with a pleasant feeling ... ... with the feeling of pride and satisfaction ... ... a feeling that you can use very well and easily feel when you leave alcohol behind ... ... because then you are proud and satisfied ... ... Choose a color for this feeling ... ... maybe blue or green or a color that you like ... ... This way you can better imagine that this feeling flows into the bottle and the level in the bottle slowly rises ... ... Just look at the image and imagine that the level in the bottle slowly rises in your desired color with the feeling of pride ... ... The empty bottle is being filled with pride ... ... the bottle that no longer contains alcohol is being filled with pride ... ... Alcohol is being replaced ... ... replaced by pride in abstaining from it ... ... Connect this with your breathing ... ... Imagine that the level in the bottle rises a bit with each inhale ... ... Every time you inhale, the level in the bottle rises because it is being filled with pride ... ... pride in your favorite color ... ... and with each exhale, you feel the relief that comes from replacing alcohol ... ... Pay attention to your body feeling because you can feel the pride with each deep inhale and the relief with each exhale ...

... ... [Speak the following suggestions always in the client's breathing rhythm. The expansion of the chest with deep inhalation is automatically associated with the body feeling of pride, and exhalation with the body feeling of relief. Sounds strange? Then observe someone telling a story with pride! Please try it!] ... ...

... ... [Client inhales] ... Inhale and let the color of pride flow into the bottle ...

... ... [Client exhales] ... and now feel the relief ... ...

... ... [Client inhales] ... Inhale and let the level of pride rise ... ...

... ... [Client exhales] ... and now feel the relief ... ...

... ... [Client inhales] ... The color of pride fills the bottle more and more ... ...

... ... [Client exhales] ... and now feel the relief ... ...

... ... [Client inhales] ... The bottle is filled only with pride ... ...

... ... [Client exhales] ... and now feel the relief ... ...

... ... [Client inhales] ... The bottle is filled only with your pride ... ...

... ... [Client exhales] ... and now feel the relief ... ...

Good ... ... very, very good ... ... Your subconscious replaces every thought of alcohol with the feeling of pride and satisfaction ... ... Whenever you think of alcohol, your subconscious immediately replaces the desire for alcohol with the feeling of pride and relief ... ... Whenever you see alcoholic beverages, your subconscious immediately replaces the desire for alcohol with the feeling of pride and relief ... ... Whenever you smell or taste alcohol, your subconscious immediately replaces the desire for alcohol with the feeling of pride and relief ... ... Whenever you think of alcohol, your subconscious immediately replaces the desire for alcohol with the feeling of pride and relief ... ... You are free from alcohol ... ... free ... ... completely free ... ...

#7

Ideomotor refers to the phenomenon that our body follows our feelings and thoughts with movements. In everyday life, this following shows as body posture, muscle tension, and movement patterns of a person, which naturally change with mood and thoughts. In trance, ideomotor signals can be used to get information that the client cannot actively communicate. For example, the subconscious can answer questions with an agreed finger signal. Of course, ideomotor reactions can also be used suggestively, for example, with arm levitation and catalepsy. Such an approach, which I also use in the following text, strengthens confidence in hypnosis and one's ability to change, thus promoting therapy.

You want to stop drinking alcohol today ... ... actually, you have already stopped, so let's deal with not starting again ... ... Perhaps it's already clear to you that it's not the alcohol that clings to you, but that you hold on to the alcohol ... ... It's almost as if you cling to it ... ... because you used to think you couldn't be without it ... ... that you needed it ... ... and possibly you even think it's inevitable ... ... Today, I want to show you that our belief often makes us hold on, even though we can let go ... ... we just need to believe that we can let go ... ... precisely when we decide to let go ... ... Maybe you're wondering how that works ... ... Maybe you want to know how I can show you that ... ... it's much easier than you think because you can show it to yourself ... ... You can convince yourself that it's only your belief that makes you hold on ... ... and if it's possible for your belief to do that, then your belief can also ensure that you can leave alcohol behind ... ... Your new belief will ensure that you leave alcohol behind ... ... and this new belief is created today because you can convince yourself of your previous error ...

... ... Imagine you couldn't do something specific, couldn't move ... ... couldn't lift your arm ... ... or couldn't open your fist ... ... You probably think now that it's not possible ... ... not opening your fist? ... ... that's not possible ... ... no, that's not possible ... ...

... [Now announce a touch and give the client a small gemstone or a coin. It should be an object that can be held well in the closed hand. Then ask the client to hold this object tightly.] ...

... ... So, let's try this thought and the feeling that goes with it ... ... I'm giving you a small stone now ... ... It's a gemstone, and you should hold it tightly ... ... Focus on your right hand and close it into a fist ... ... Imagine you have to hold the stone so tightly that no one can open your fist against your will ... ... You close your fist tighter and tighter ... ... very tight ... ... Your fist becomes tighter and tighter ... ... No one can take this stone from you ... ... no one can open your fist ... ... Nothing and no one can open your fist now because you close it tighter and tighter ... ... and at the thought of having to open it, you close it even tighter because you won't let anything be taken away from you ... ... As soon as someone tries to open your fist, you close it even tighter ... ... As soon as anyone tries to open your fist, it automatically closes even tighter than now ... ... Whoever tries to open your fist, it closes tighter ... ... exactly so ... ... that's right ... ... If I were to try to open your fist now ...

... [Now announce a touch and try with little force to open the client's fist. Please do not use force, it should not succeed. The client should show an impulse to close the fist tighter.] ...

... ... Your fist closes tighter ... ... You close your fist ... ... Excellent ... ... You imprint this deeply ... ... the attempt to open your fist closes it even tighter ... ... Even if you now tried to stretch your fingers, your fist closes tighter ... ... Try to stretch your fingers, and your fist closes ...

... [If the fingers do open a little, follow up with a suggestion ... Your fist closes, yes, your fist closes ...] ...

... ... It doesn't work anymore ... ... your fist can't be opened anymore, but why? ... ... Because you believe it ... ... If you believed you could open it, it would succeed ... ... Imagine your fingers were made of rubber ... ... very flexible and soft ... ... very flexible and soft, and imagine that you decide to move your flexible fingers and above all ... ... want to move them ... ... Then your fingers loosen, relax ... ... just like that ... ... You can open your hand because you can relax it ... ... because you want to ... ... Open your hand loosely and let the stone fall ... ... Just let the stone fall ... ... just like that ... ... It succeeds ... ... Move your fingers and check that you can actually move them well again ... ... Now allow yourself to rest and follow a special thought ... ... It's the thought that explains to you that your belief in needing alcohol is just like the belief in an unopenable hand ... ... You can always do exactly what you believe ... ... and if you believe you can let go of alcohol, then you can let go of it ... ... simply let go ... ... Alcohol then falls away from you, just like the gemstone fell to the ground ...

... ... Your inner self deeply imprints that you are now free and can go new ways ... ... and whenever you want to remember that you can let go of everything you want to get rid of, you simply take the gemstone in your hand, close your fist briefly, and open it again because you decide what you let go of ... ... You carry this stone with you for the next few weeks because it is a signal and reminder for you that only your belief decides what can be ... ... and with every thought of drinking, you take the stone in your hand, close your fist, and open it again, and the thought passes ...

#8

The following hypnosis works with the connection between emotion and body. Since all feelings, as well as thoughts, show in physical reactions, sometimes clearly, often also very subtly, focusing on body perceptions and attentively paying attention to body signals can help in solving problems. The client should be able to physically feel their deep emotions and thus react more quickly to signs of emotional change. Suggestive techniques help influence body sensations to change emotions, as not only feelings create physical reactions, but deliberate body use also affects emotions. Joy, for example, creates a smile; conversely, a deliberate smile also tends to brighten the mood.

In this hypnosis, the client should place a hand on their body, somewhat in the liver area. Discuss with your client beforehand where and how they can place a hand there. Not everyone knows where the liver is!

You are here today to free yourself even more from alcohol ... ... You have already decided to abstain from alcohol, and you have already realized that it's not really a renunciation ... ... because you gain much more than you could ever give up ... ... You gain freedom ... ... You gain health ... ... and you gain a much more pleasant and better body feeling ... ... Today, you can work specifically with your body feeling and accomplish two special things ... ... On the one hand, you can improve your body feeling, feel your body, and learn to pay attention to and listen to its striving for health ... ... But you can do much more ... ... You can help your body become completely free ... ... free from alcohol ... ... even freer than before ... ... because your body can develop this feeling of completely rejecting alcohol ... ... with your help, your body can become an absolute anti-alcohol person ... ... It's easier than you think ... ... It's about the connection between thoughts and body feeling ... ... Maybe you think that's always the case anyway, that body and thoughts always form a unit ... ... But in the past, you often misunderstood and thought your body wanted alcohol ... ... but that's not true ... ... Your thoughts thought that, and your body only reacted to it ... ... Today, you can ensure that your body rejects alcohol ... ... So let's begin to show your body that you really don't need or want alcohol anymore ...

... ... Pay attention to your body feeling now ... ... your body can feel very pleasant and good now ... ... it probably feels good because you are relaxed now ... ... If you want to feel even more comfortable, just make yourself more comfortable ... ... as comfortable as possible ... ... [If the client moves, wait until they are comfortable and calm again] ... ... good ... ... and now place a hand on your body, somewhat where your liver is ... ... The liver has experienced the most ... ... It has endured the burdens of alcohol the most ... ... So it is the center of change ... ... You now place your protective and helping hand on your liver ... ... Feel the warmth that comes from your hand and your body ... ... That's where your liver is ... ... That's where the alcohol and the thought of drinking are ... ... All our feelings and needs, all our thoughts are stored somewhere in our body, showing as a feeling ... ... and your thoughts of drinking are located where your hand is now ... ... your protective hand, because you protect your liver and your body from further attacks by alcohol ... ... You have already decided not to drink alcohol anymore ... ... and now the old need for alcohol can also go because you don't need it anymore ... ... It can dissolve now in the warmth of your protective hand ... ... Perhaps you can already feel the change in the warmth ... ... maybe you can already feel in your body that the old drinking pattern is dissolving ... ... and dissolving in the warmth ... ... The old need for alcohol is slowly dissolving in the warmth of your protective hand ... ... Focus entirely on the feeling between your protective hand and your body ... ... The old need for alcohol is slowly dissolving in the warmth of your protective hand ... ... Breathe deeply in and out and feel deeply into your body ... ... and the old need for alcohol is dissolving in the warmth of your own hand ... ... because your will to never drink alcohol again is your most important thought ... ... and your most important thought flows into your hand ... ... your own hand takes over this thought because you know that the body can always feel what is in your thoughts if you pay attention to the connection between body and thoughts ... ... and now you are paying special attention to it ... ... Your hand takes over this thought and this will ... ... Your hand wants to banish alcohol ... ... Your hand wants to protect you from alcohol ... ... Your hand wants to protect your body from alcohol ... ... your hand wants to protect your liver from alcohol, which quietly dissolves everything related to alcohol ... ... now, at this moment, while you hear my voice, your liver frees itself from alcohol and builds a completely new body feeling ... ... a completely new need for healthy and fresh drinks ... ... With fresh water, you can soon cleanse your body ... ... Your body develops a strong need for fresh water under the protection of your hand ... ... and whenever you might think of drinking alcohol, your body signals a strong need for fresh water ... ... Your protective hand almost eliminates alcohol because your body completely rejects alcohol ... ... Your protective hand helps your body now to banish alcohol ... ... to banish alcohol forever ... ... Feel deeply into your body and recognize that your body completely adjusts and becomes an anti-drinker ... ... free from alcohol ...

... ... You feel the change in your body and make it clear that your body, with the help of your protective hand, banishes alcohol forever ... ... So, every day you pay attention to your body and take five minutes in the morning after waking up and place your protective hand on your liver ... ... so you remind yourself that you never want to drink again, and you give your body the signal that you will really take care of its well-being and health on this day ... ... and whenever you place your hand on your liver, you can distance yourself even more from alcohol, and your body helps you reject alcohol immediately and supports you in leading a healthy life ...

#9

Today we embark on a journey together ... ... a journey only possible because you can sink deeply into your thoughts ... ... dive into your imagination and find yourself deep in your imagination ... ... In your dreams, you can imagine everything, even what seems impossible ... ... But most of the time, much more is possible than we believe because imagination and reality are very close together, sometimes even the same ... ... and when the right moment comes, any daydream can become a beautiful truth ... ... and who knows, maybe the right moment is now ... ... right now, at this exact moment ... ... so you direct your attention and mindfulness to the center of your body, where your gut feeling also resides, and imagine you could sink entirely into this point ... ... sink deeper and deeper into yourself to be completely in your feeling ... ... to arrive now in the land of your dreams ...

... ... You stand in a beautiful garden where everything is in bloom ... ... blooming bushes and climbing roses adorn this lovely garden, inviting you to go deeper and find a special place ... ... Deep in your imagination, there are only special places because every place can always be a part of you and show you something of yourself ... ... and everything you are is special ... ... unique and above all always in motion ... ... How often in life do we believe there is no progress, that we are condemned to stand still and be stuck in our problems ... ... But there is always the possibility of constructive change ... ... Sometimes we just need to understand what keeps us standing still ... ... You have often sought refuge in alcohol, feeling that everything was lost or that you couldn't bear the problems anymore ... ... and if you think about why you sought refuge in alcohol today, you don't know exactly ... ... Maybe it just happened, and you noticed it late ... ... but not too late because you are now in the garden to do something ... ... to understand what's behind

the alcohol ... ... You follow a narrow path leading you through the garden ... ... You walk under rose arches, like through a tunnel guiding you ... ... and then you arrive at a place of peace and reflection ... ... a round place in the middle of the garden, so deep inside that it cannot be seen from the outside ... ... no one can look in here except you ...

... In the center of the round place of peace and reflection, there is a stone well ... ... and on the wall of the well stands a jug ... ... You look around and see the colorful splendor of the many flowers and plants in the garden ... ... and suddenly you smell alcohol ... ... Then you think about what actually drove you to drink ... ... a feeling that drove you ... ... maybe loneliness or fear ... ... perhaps unfulfilled love or longing ... ... or grief and pain ... ... there is something behind the alcohol that you couldn't deal with because you didn't even know it was about that ... ... Today you can and will find an answer to this question ... ... because in the land of dreams, every answer awaits you ... ... everything is here ... ... every truth is here ... ... So you walk across the place in the depth and follow the smell of alcohol ... ... It comes from the well ... ... You go to the well, which is filled to the top with clear and fresh water ... ... You scoop a handful of water from the well and drink it, and it is indeed water ... ... pure water ... ... Then you look at the jug standing on the wall of the well ... ... You smell it and realize that this jug is filled with alcohol ... ... But you don't want to drink alcohol anymore and pour it out, you simply pour the alcohol onto the ground and set the jug down again ... ... but it is filled with alcohol again … … as if by magic, it fills with alcohol … … So you try again to empty it, but again it does not succeed … … What is special about this jug? Why does it refill itself? … … There is no hose filling it, it is just a normal jug, but something at the bottom of the jug ensures it always refills … … So you look through the alcohol to the bottom of the jug … … Your gaze goes deeper and deeper … … and the deeper your gaze sinks into the alcohol jug, the more clearly you can feel your body feeling, the more clearly you can feel your mood … … feel your feelings … … and at the bottom of the jug, an image slowly emerges … … slowly colors and shapes appear, and soon images … … Or perhaps a specific image that shows you why you started with alcohol … … The image at the bottom of the jug shows you how it once began … … and slowly this image rises, whatever it is … … The image slowly rises from the depth of the jug and swims through the alcohol to the surface … … You look at it, but more important than this image is your feeling … … because with every image in us, we connect a feeling … … and it is the feeling in this image that made you start drinking … … Back then, it had to happen that way, you couldn't react any other way because the time wasn't right … … but today it's different … … today you can learn from this image how to avoid alcohol … … how to refrain from drinking because you can also deal with your feelings differently … … even painful feelings you can endure … … if you allow them, they can also pass … … Now you see the image, and now it is time to pour out the alcohol because you know the image and feel your feeling …

So you pour out the jug and set it down again … … it remains empty because you are now ready to accept the images and feelings at the bottom of the jug and deal with them … … without alcohol … … You rinse out the jug … … Then you fill it with fresh water and take a big sip of the pure water … … Then you think about the fact that the land of dreams is deep within you … … It has always been there … … I'm just telling you about it …

#10

Imagination has no limits, only those we impose on ourselves ... ... But there are no boundaries that can stop us in imagination ... ... You know the song "Die Gedanken sind frei" and that means that imagination is also free ... ... So I invite you to a journey in your imagination ... ... Everything you can imagine there can also happen ... ... What is possible there can also become reality ... ... and deep in your imagination, in your dreams, you can let go of alcohol today ... ... So imagine you could leave your body and float away like the wind to embark on a journey to a very special land ... ... a land of liberation and renewal ... ... a land of truly unlimited and fantastic possibilities ... ... the land of dreams ... ... With the next breath, you are there ...

You stand in a field of sunflowers, in the middle of the tall flowers that shine so brightly and smell wonderfully ... ... You walk between the long stems of the sunflowers and follow your feeling, the best compass you can ever have ... ... You find a sphere that looks like a giant soap bubble, so big that you can go inside ... ... You go into this sphere and stand in a dense fog ... ... You hear a laugh, a cheeky grin ... ... You think, What is this? and then you hear a voice from the fog ... ... It says: You are in the bubble of alcohol ... ... in the bubble of your addiction ... ... Come closer ... ... Your addiction is here ... ... The fog slowly clears, and you see a dark figure before you ... ... A person cloaked in a dark robe ... ... They wear a hood and have no face ... ... It looks as if this mysterious figure has no head ... ... You ask: Who are you? What do you want from me? ... ... The dark figure answers: I am your addiction, your craving for alcohol ... ... I have been waiting here for you for a very long time ... ... I have been handling some of your tasks for so long ... ... The figure explains why it is here ... ... It says: Even if you didn't know it. I often help you ... ... For example, I allow you to give up responsibility ... ... Sometimes you can avoid confrontations because of me ... ... You can withdraw and block out all the strenuous things ... ... Often this bothers you ... ... But sometimes you also had advantages from it, if you think about it carefully ... ... You try to fight against me ... ... I will show you who you are fighting against ... ... The dark figure pulls back the hood and shows its face ... ... You recognize that the person hidden behind the dark cloak looks exactly like you ... ... As if you were looking in a mirror ... ... I am part of you ... ... I am your addiction ... ... I am you ... ... I am you ... ... You stand facing this person and recognize yourself ... ... At this moment, you understand that you are fighting against yourself when you fight against your addiction ... ... So you ask this mysterious person standing before you what you can do to finally let go of alcohol without fighting against yourself ... ... Your counterpart says: I am only here until you understand that I am part of you and have a function ... ... If you can accept that and realize that you are not my victim but my reflection, I will leave ... ... But even if you cannot find anything helpful in me, it is enough to acknowledge my significance ... ... Give me your hand as a sign of acceptance ... ... You approach this person in the bubble ... ... They are your reflection, you are yourself ... ... The addiction is part of you ... ... You reach out your hand to this part, like a helping hand ... ... You make it clear that you are extending your hand to your addiction and thereby to yourself ... ... When you are ready, extend your hand to this part of you now ... ... You feel this connection. You feel that everything you fought against was a part of you ... ... And even this part of you was important ... ... It made you aware and helped you take this step today ... ... The step of letting go ... ... Now you can let go of so much and build new things ... ... You let go of drinking and rebuild your strength for confrontation and conflict resolution ... ... You rebuild your self-confidence and your joy of life ... ... And while you think about all this, you continue to hold the hand of your reflection as a sign that you are ready to recognize and accept all this as parts of yourself ... ... And the figure in the dark cloak, which was a part of you, crumbles into white dust because you no longer need this part ... ... You understood the addiction, you know it was a part of you ... ... Now it is time for renewal ... ... What you need is a fresh breeze ... ... and suddenly a warm wind blows through the bubble you are standing in ... ... and carries away the white dust ... ... You feel free ... ... You feel free now ... ... You leave the bubble ... ... You are standing again in the sunflower field, the flowers bowing towards you ... ... You continue to walk through the field, and the flowers move aside to make your path easier ... ... Once more you turn around and see the bubble gently burst like a soap bubble in the wind ... ... You make it clear to yourself that you can encounter everything you are in a bubble again ...

... Every day, if you want, or whenever problems arise deep within you ... ... Again and again, you can extend your hand to your inner parts and make peace with them ... ... They then crumble into white dust, carried away by the wind ... ... And you feel freer ...

You feel the feeling of liberation and relief deep within you ... ... and you can see the fine white dust carried by the wind across the field ... ... The white dust becomes fertilizer for the growth of new flowers because every constructive change creates the basis for new growth ... ... Here in the land of dreams, everything is possible, including the liberation

from alcohol ... ... including the rediscovery of your own strength and self-confidence, which now take the place that was previously occupied by alcohol ... ... Self-confidence replaces alcohol ... ... now ... ... Self-confidence replaces alcohol ... ... now ... ... Then you think about the fact that the land of dreams is deep within you ... ... It has always been there ... ... I'm just telling you about it ...

Distribution, publication, and copying in any form are prohibited and subject to damages.

Overview of All Titles in the Series "Ten Hypnoses"

Volume 1: Smoking Cessation
Volume 2: Anxiety and Restlessness
Volume 3: Burnout
Volume 4: Reducing Overweight
Volume 5: Coping with the Past
Volume 6: Suicidal Thoughts and Attempts
Volume 7: Psycho-Oncology
Volume 8: Obsessions and Tics
Volume 9: Self-Confidence and Decision-Making
Volume 10: Grief Work
Volume 11: Psychosomatics
Volume 12: Chronic Pain
Volume 13: Depressive Thoughts
Volume 14: Panic Attacks
Volume 15: Domestic Violence, Victim Support
Volume 16: Post-Traumatic Stress
Volume 17: Exam Anxiety and Stage Fright
Volume 18: Anti-Violence Training, Offender Support
Volume 19: Addiction Tendencies
Volume 20: Social Phobia and Fear of Contact
Volume 21: Nail Biting
Volume 22: Self-Awareness and Self-Love
Volume 23: Teeth Grinding and Night Clenching
Volume 24: Feelings of Guilt
Volume 25: Fear in Crowds
Volume 26: Fear of Flying, Aviophobia
Volume 27: Fear in Enclosed Spaces, Claustrophobia
Volume 28: Tinnitus, Ear Noises
Volume 29: Fear of Heights
Volume 30: Neurodermatitis

Copying, publishing, and sharing with third parties are only permitted with the written consent of the author. Please observe the notes on copyright and usage.

Volume 31: Finding Inner Balance
Volume 32: Overcoming Loneliness
Volume 33: Fear of Illness, Hypochondria
Volume 34: Anticipatory Anxiety, Fear of Fear
Volume 35: Jealousy in Relationships
Volume 36: Driving Anxiety
Volume 37: New Start after Separation
Volume 38: Fear of Injections
Volume 39: Heart Anxiety Neurosis
Volume 40: Overcoming Resentment and Anger
Volume 41: Resolving Blockages and Positive Thinking
Volume 42: Stress Reduction, Stress Management
Volume 43: Body Relaxation
Volume 44: Deep Relaxation
Volume 45: Fear of the Dark
Volume 46: Falling Asleep and Staying Asleep
Volume 47: Compulsive Buying
Volume 48: Restless Legs Syndrome
Volume 49: Bulimia
Volume 50: Anorexia
Volume 51: Overcoming Nightmares
Volume 52: Imagined Deformity
Volume 53: Overcoming Distrust, Finding Trust
Volume 54: Processing Failures
Volume 55: Humiliation, Emotional Hurt
Volume 56: Distressing Compassion, Vicarious Suffering
Volume 57: Self-Forgiveness
Volume 58: Self-Awareness, Self-Confidence
Volume 59: Saying No
Volume 60: Assertiveness
Volume 61: Setting Boundaries and Self-Assertion
Volume 62: Decision-Making Ability

Volume 63: Success Orientation
Volume 64: Ruminating, Circular Thinking
Volume 65: Accepting Pregnancy
Volume 66: Birth Preparation
Volume 67: Spiritual Opening
Volume 68: Joy of Life and Inner Lightness
Volume 69: Patience and Inner Peace
Volume 70: Fibromyalgia and Rheumatism
Volume 71: Irritable Bowel Syndrome, Crohn's Disease
Volume 72: Fear of Nausea, Emetophobia
Volume 73: Stuttering and Cluttering, Speech Flow Disorders
Volume 74: Concentration and Knowledge Anchoring
Volume 75: Vitality and Spontaneity
Volume 76: Searching for Meaning and Finding Goals
Volume 77: Life Crises, Life Events
Volume 78: Workaholism, Goal Obsession
Volume 79: Helper Syndrome, Helpless Helpers
Volume 80: Medication Abuse
Volume 81: Gambling Addiction
Volume 82: Internet Addiction, Smartphone Addiction
Volume 83: Hoarding Disorder, Compulsive Collecting
Volume 84: Conspiracy Thoughts, Overvalued Ideas
Volume 85: Fear of Operations and Treatments
Volume 86: Fear of Aging
Volume 87: Travel Anxiety
Volume 88: Anxiety When Urinating, Paruresis
Volume 89: Fear of Intimacy and Togetherness
Volume 90: Fear of Blushing
Volume 91: Coming Out in Homosexuality
Volume 92: Charisma Training
Volume 93: Migraines and Chronic Headaches
Volume 94: Overcoming Allergies, Bronchial Asthma

Volume 95: Normalizing Blood Pressure
Volume 96: Compulsive Perfectionism
Volume 97: Sports Hypnosis, Motivation
Volume 98: Sports Hypnosis, Performance Enhancement
Volume 99: Determination and Focus
Volume 100: Encountering the Inner Child
Volume 101: Cravings, Binge Eating
Volume 102: Stimulating Metabolism
Volume 103: Bipolar Mood Swings
Volume 104: Borderline, Identity Crises
Volume 105: Hypomania, Euphoria, Mania
Volume 106: Restlessness, Agitation
Volume 107: Nervous Breakdown
Volume 108: Adjustment Disorders
Volume 109: Self-Alienation, Depersonalization
Volume 110: Ending Self-Pity
Volume 111: Primary Gain of Illness
Volume 112: Secondary Gain of Illness
Volume 113: Bullying, Victim Support
Volume 114: Letting Go of Envy and Jealousy
Volume 115: Fear of Spiders, Arachnophobia
Volume 116: Fear of Dogs or Cats
Volume 117: Fear of Strangers, Xenophobia
Volume 118: Excessive Worries, Generalized Anxiety
Volume 119: Strengthening Sense of Responsibility
Volume 120: Unrequited Love, Heartache
Volume 121: Work-Life Balance
Volume 122: Letting Go of Unattainable Goals
Volume 123: Allowing and Accepting Help
Volume 124: Letting Go of Adult Children
Volume 125: Tourette Syndrome
Volume 126: Life Changes and New Starts

Volume 127: Accepting Life in a Wheelchair
Volume 128: Understanding and Overcoming Homesickness
Volume 129: Understanding and Overcoming Wanderlust
Volume 130: Dizziness, Meniere's Disease
Volume 131: Overcoming Aggression
Volume 132: Cutting and Self-Harm
Volume 133: Hair Pulling, Trichotillomania
Volume 134: Postpartum Depression
Volume 135: For Relatives of Dementia Patients
Volume 136: Self-Harm, Artificial Disorders
Volume 137: Activating Self-Healing Powers
Volume 138: Preventing Depression Relapse
Volume 139: Reactive Psychoses, Follow-Up
Volume 140: Obsessive Thoughts and Impulses
Volume 141: Compulsive Checking
Volume 142: Compulsive Counting, Symmetry Obsession
Volume 143: Compulsive Washing, Cleanliness Obsession
Volume 144: Compulsive Questioning
Volume 145: Dissociative Paralysis
Volume 146: Phantom Pain
Volume 147: Overcoming Complaining
Volume 148: Hay Fever, Pollen Allergy
Volume 149: Sexual Abuse, Victim Support
Volume 150: Standing Strong Against Sexism, #metoo
Volume 151: Binge Eating
Volume 152: Overcoming Thoughts of Revenge
Volume 153: Detachment from the Aggressor, Stockholm Syndrome
Volume 154: Courage to Separate
Volume 155: Chronic Fatigue, Exhaustion
Volume 156: Fear of the Future, Existential Anxiety
Volume 157: Excessive Worry About Children
Volume 158: Fear of Failure

Volume 159: Ending Distrust and Control
Volume 160: Dejection, Dysphoria
Volume 161: Boreout, Chronic Boredom
Volume 162: Bipolar Disorders, Relapse Prevention
Volume 163: Mania, Relapse Prevention
Volume 164: Nihilism, Feelings of Worthlessness
Volume 165: Thumb Sucking
Volume 166: Being Brave
Volume 167: Being Proud
Volume 168: Overcoming Shyness
Volume 169: Being Able to Delegate Responsibility
Volume 170: Being Able to Show Emotions
Volume 171: Letting Go of Guilt, Victim Support
Volume 172: Processing Guilt, Offender Support
Volume 173: Mood Swings, Cyclothymia
Volume 174: Lack of Drive, Vital Sadness
Volume 175: Hearing Voices with Reality Reference
Volume 176: Confident Communication
Volume 177: Standing Up for Oneself
Volume 178: Taking New Paths
Volume 179: Confident Job Application
Volume 180: No Longer Being Taken Advantage Of
Volume 181: End of Submissiveness
Volume 182: Depressive Numbness
Volume 183: Mood Drops, Affective Incontinence
Volume 184: Mood Instability
Volume 185: Somatoform Disorders
Volume 186: Stomach Ulcer, Psychosomatic
Volume 187: Accepting Amputation
Volume 188: Overcoming and Letting Go of Hatred
Volume 189: Ending Accusations
Volume 190: Allowing Tears, Being Able to Cry

Volume 191: Finding and Sorting Repressed Feelings
Volume 192: Somatoform Pain
Volume 193: Living Autonomously
Volume 194: Anhedonia, Joylessness
Volume 195: Persistent Sadness
Volume 196: Obesity, Food Addiction
Volume 197: Parents of Abused Children
Volume 198: Letting Go and Letting Be
Volume 199: Childhood Sexual Abuse
Volume 200: Fear of Loss

www.ingramcontent.com/pod-product-compliance
Lightning Source LLC
Chambersburg PA
CBHW030456220526
45464CB00006B/2554